The Anemia Cure

Dr. Susan's Healthy Living
drsusanshealthyliving.com

Facebook.com/DrSusanRichards
drsusanshealthyliving@gmail.com
(650) 561-9978

Mention of specific companies or products in this book does not suggest endorsement by the author or publisher. Internet addresses and telephone numbers for resources provided in this book were accurate at the time it went to press.

ISBN 978-1512226706

Note

The information in this book is meant to complement the advice and guidance of your physician, not replace it. It is very important that any person who has medical problems be evaluated by a physician. If you are under the care of a physician, you should discuss any major changes in your regimen with him or her. Because this is a book and not a medical consultation, keep in mind that the information presented here may not apply in your particular case. In view of individual medical requirements, new research, and government regulations, it is the responsibility of the reader to validate health practices and treatments with a physician or health service.

Table of Contents

Introduction

Dear Friend,

I am thrilled that you have found my book, *The Anemia Cure* because I know that you are looking for positive and effective solutions for anemia. I have written this book just for you, to share with you the all-natural treatment program that I have developed and successfully treated thousands of my patients.

Anemia is a very common issue that millions of women suffer from. While in women, anemia is primarily due to menstrual bleeding, it can also be related to intestinal bleeding, poor blood formation and other causes. Anemia can often easily be treated and prevented. I have written this book to share with you the most effective and helpful self-care treatments for this issue.

My Self-Care Approach To Anemia

In my medical practice, I have always combined self-care treatments along with any medical therapies. After seeing so many of my patients become healed from this issue, I am a firm believer in the power of self-care. Changing your lifestyle habits in beneficial ways gives your body the chance to heal itself. My goal as a physician is to help my patients become symptom-free, thereby reducing their need for medical care. I don't believe that an unfavorable medical diagnosis need be a lifetime sentence of poor health.

In working with my anemia patients, I have not only corrected the anemia itself but also the underlying imbalances that were causing this problem in the first place. Anemia is commonly seen in women in their thirties, forties and early fifties as a consequence of estrogen dominant related conditions like fibroid tumors, endometriosis, polyps and other conditions. The hormonal imbalances related to estrogen dominance need to be corrected so the excessive blood loss and resulting anemia are eliminated. Pregnant women also frequently become anemic due to the expansion of the blood volume that takes place during this time as well as their increased nutritional needs. Some women become anemic due to blood loss from the digestive tract due to endometriosis and other conditions.

How to Use This Book

This anemia self-care program provides very important information for all women suffering from anemia. I discuss in much greater detail than you will ever receive during a routine medical visit with your doctor the nutritional factors that are necessary for healthy blood formation. Most women are just treated with iron replacement, however healthy blood formation requires a variety of essential nutrients.

I have also included great meal plans and recipes with this book that will support healthy balanced hormones to help eliminate the causes of bleeding as well as support healthy blood formation

This program is practical and easy to follow. It can be used by itself or in conjunction with a medical program. And best of all, it works. I look forward to you reading and benefitting from this book for the treatment of anemia.

Love,

Dr. Susan

Part I:
Learning About the Problem

1

What Is Anemia?

I want to start this book by sharing with you much important information about anemia. You will be learning about how your red blood cells are formed, how anemia occurs as well as its symptoms and risk factors. I also discuss how anemia is diagnosed. This helpful information will set a strong foundation for you that will enable you to better correct this issue.

Anemia is one of the most common health problems affecting women of all ages. It has been estimated that as many as 20 percent of all American women suffer from anemia. Anemia can be found in all age groups—from childhood to old age. It is not restricted in frequency to any one period of a woman's life. Anemia is characterized by a reduction in the number of red blood cells or a reduction in hemoglobin (the oxygen-carrying protein in red blood cells).

Anemia reduces the amount of oxygen available to all cells of the body; then, carbon dioxide, a waste product, accumulates in the cells and cannot be removed by the lungs with normal respirations. As a result of the blood's lower oxygen-carrying capability, the cells for the body's normal chemical functioning have less available energy. Important processes, such as muscular activity, and cell building and repair, slow down and become less efficient. Greater than 95 percent of the body's chemical reactions depend on optimal oxygen levels in cells and tissues. As a result, the symptoms of anemia can be very debilitating.

The Symptoms

The symptoms of anemia are numerous and affect many organ systems in the body. Often the symptoms seem vague and misleading to women and to their physicians. In fact, every symptom of anemia can be mistaken for other health conditions, including nervous tension and emotional problems. Because the lack of oxygen impairs the body's ability to carry out its numerous chemical reactions, many women with anemia feel extremely tired and fatigued. Because muscular activity is inhibited, they lack endurance and physical stamina. I have had many physically active patients who had to stop pursuing vigorous aerobic exercise programs when they developed anemia. These women simply lacked the physical energy to continue their active exercise regimens once the anemia became too severe.

When the brain cells lack oxygen, dizziness may result and mental faculties are less sharp. Women who are anemic tend to be pale with poor skin color and tone. They often appear "washed-out" and seem listless. They lack the glowing skin color that we tend to associate with good health and vitality. Women with anemia may also suffer from hair loss and brittle, ridged fingernails.

Digestive symptoms include loss of appetite, sore tongue, abdominal pain, heartburn, and diarrhea. In more severe cases, women can suffer from symptoms as varied as headaches, heart palpitations, tingling in the fingers and feet, loss of coordination, and a yellowing of the skin. As you can see, a woman can become quite ill from the physical and mental effects of anemia if her physician does not diagnose her condition properly.

Symptoms of Anemia

General weakness	Loss of coordination	Brittle and ridged nails
Fatigue	Loss of appetite	Yellowing of skin
Dizziness	Abdominal pain	Tingling in hands and
Paleness	Sore tongue	feet
Diarrhea		

How Red Blood Cells Are Formed

To understand anemia, you should first understand how normal red blood cells are produced. Then you can follow how the different types of anemia occur, particularly those due to nutritional deficiencies in which a lack of proper nutrients impairs the normal production of red blood cells.

Before birth, as we grow and mature in the uterus, our bodies have no specific centers for red cell production. Red cells are formed in many places: the yolk sac, spleen, liver, thymus gland, lymph nodes, and bone marrow. After birth and as we grow toward adulthood, the production of red cells shifts predominantly to the red bone marrow of certain bones, including the pelvis, vertebrae, ribs, sternum or chest bone, skull, and the humerus and femur (the bones of arms and legs).

The formation of new, immature red cells takes place in the bone marrow. The immature red cells go through several transformations before gaining the ability to produce hemoglobin, the oxygen-carrying protein found in red blood cells. After several more transformations in the bone marrow, the red blood cells mature to cells called reticulocytes. Reticulocytes contain about one-third of their weight in hemoglobin. At maturity, red blood cells lose their nuclei, or core; this transformation makes the cells more fluid and flexible. With this increased flexibility, the reticulocytes can leave the bone marrow and enter the bloodstream by squeezing through the walls of the small blood vessels or capillaries.

The mature red blood cell looks like a concave disk on both sides and has a very simple structure with no core or nucleus. It also lacks the ability to reproduce or carry on extensive chemical activities. The red blood cell has an outer cell membrane composed of protein that encloses the cell body (or cytoplasm) and the hemoglobin. The hemoglobin molecule consists of a protein called globin and a pigment called heme, which contains iron. Hemoglobin is a red-colored pigment that is responsible for the red color of the blood.

As mentioned earlier, the hemoglobin allows the oxygen to attach to the red blood cells and be transported throughout the body. A healthy woman has about 4.7 million red blood cells per cubic millimeter of blood (a very small unit of volume), while a healthy man has about 5.4 million red blood cells per cubic millimeter of blood.

Since the life span of a red blood cell is only 120 days, the body constantly breaks down old red blood cells and forms new ones. In fact, the body produces an astonishing 2 million new red blood cells per second. The old red blood cells are destroyed in the liver and spleen, and these substances are either reused or eliminated from the body. If this process breaks down at any point, then anemia, or lack of red blood cells, can occur.

How Anemia Is Diagnosed

Health-care providers can diagnose anemia simply by removing a small sample of blood from the body and looking at the characteristics and number of red blood cells. This is one of the most common medical tests done on patients in the United States. When evaluating the blood sample for anemia, the total number of red blood cells is counted. The percentage of blood that is made up of red blood cells, or the hematocrit, is also estimated by determining the ratio of red blood cells to the whole blood.

In healthy women the hematocrit averages 38 to 47 percent; it is lower in women with anemia. In this blood test, the hemoglobin level, or amount of pigment in the blood, is commonly estimated also. For healthy women, the normal range is 12.0 to 15.0 grams per deciliter.

Hemoglobin level, red blood cells, and hematocrit are all reduced in women with anemia. Specific deficiencies of nutrients related to anemia can also be measured. With iron-deficiency anemia, blood iron levels are decreased, iron binding capacity is increased, and the iron saturation transferrin (a protein that binds iron) is decreased.

Blood tests for the other nutrient deficiencies associated with anemia (such as vitamin B12 and folic acid) are also available. Normal levels of B12 are 200 to 400 mcg per ml and for folic acid are 7 or more nanograms per ml.

Causes of Anemia

The most common cause of anemia is iron deficiency. When women are iron-deficient, their red blood cells do not mature properly and remain small and pale-colored. It has been estimated that as many as one-third to one-half of young American women have low or depleted iron stores. The main reason for these low reserves is that women simply don't eat enough iron-rich foods. Many women diet excessively, so their total caloric intake does not contain sufficient foods to sustain an adequate iron reserve.

For some women, dairy products such as yogurt, cheese, and cottage cheese constitute their main source of protein. Dairy products are very low in iron content. Women who eat a lot of "junk foods" such as candy bars, chocolate, french fries, and other high-fat, high-sugar foods are also stacking their dietary intake toward inadequate amounts of iron. Women athletes also have an increased need for iron during training because of the metabolic demands of heavy exercise.

Children, adolescents, and women during their reproductive years require adequate iron. This iron is needed to support growth and development in children and teenage girls and to replace the iron lost in the monthly menstrual period during a woman's reproductive years. During an average menstrual period, it is estimated a woman loses approximately 18 mg of iron through the loss of red blood cells. This equals a daily average iron loss of 0.6 mg over a month's time.

As a result, women during their reproductive years need twice as much iron intake as men. This need persists until menopause, when the monthly blood loss finally ceases. Elderly women are still susceptible to developing anemia because they tend to eat less and have a nutrient-poor diet, which may be due to living alone or having a limited income.

Pregnancy and the postpartum period are vulnerable times for women. During pregnancy, the volume of the mother's blood increases and the growing fetus has its own needs for iron. To meet these demands, pregnant women must increase their iron intake through proper dietary habits as well as iron supplementation. Nursing mothers need iron to build up the reserves that were depleted during pregnancy. Also, iron is lost through the breast milk because this important mineral is used to fortify the newborn infant and must be replaced by the lactating mother.

The official recommendations for iron intake at all phases of a woman's life are as follows:

Pregnant women	30 mg per day
Nursing mothers	15 mg per day
Teenagers through reproductive years	15 mg per day
Postmenopausal women	10 mg per day

Besides consuming an adequate amount of iron in your diet, you must also be able to absorb the iron properly. Even if you have an iron-rich diet, the lack of vitamin A or of B vitamins such as thiamine (B1), riboflavin (B2), niacin (B3), and pantothenic acid (B5) can result in an under- or non-absorption of iron. Iron absorption is also decreased by chronic diarrhea, laxative abuse, and malabsorption diseases such as celiac disease and sprue. Vitamin C can be very helpful in facilitating iron absorption. At least 75 mg must be provided daily in the diet, either through a combination of fruits and vegetables or the use of a supplement. However, you should avoid calcium supplements and calcium carbonate-based antacids when you ingest iron supplements or iron-rich foods, because calcium inhibits iron absorption.

Another common reason for the development of iron deficiency anemia is excessive blood loss, such as that experienced by women who suffer from menorrhagia (heavy or prolonged menstrual bleeding). Menorrhagia is commonly seen in women with problems such as hormonal imbalances, fibroid tumors, and uterine cancer. Women who use intrauterine devices for contraception are also at higher risk of blood loss. In fact, it is estimated that 10 percent of women using IUDs have significant loss of blood, and therefore iron. The excessive use of anti-inflammatory medications such as aspirin or ibuprofen can cause blood loss through the digestive tract. This occurs because anti-inflammatory medication causes irritation of the stomach lining.

Iron is not the only mineral needed for healthy red blood cell production. Two other minerals, copper and zinc, also play important roles. Copper assists in the formation of hemoglobin and red blood cells by increasing iron absorption. Zinc deficiency has been found in people suffering from sickle-cell anemia. Clinical studies have shown that zinc supplementation helped decrease the number of sickled cells.

Pernicious anemia is another form of anemia caused by nutritional deficiencies, in this case, vitamin B12. This deficiency can often be traced to the inability of the stomach to secrete the "intrinsic factor" a substance necessary for the absorption of vitamin B12. The lack of the intrinsic factor is an inherited trait and results in a severe form of anemia in which the red blood cells do not grow and mature properly. People of European ancestry are more likely to inherit this trait. Women who suffer from inflammatory diseases of the small intestine, such as Crohn's disease or ilietis, run a higher risk of B12 deficiency because of their inability to absorb it through the small intestine.

The symptoms of vitamin B12 deficiency can be slow to appear once the body's supply of this nutrient diminishes, usually taking as long as four to six years once B12 stores are depleted. As a result of B12 deficiency, the body produces fewer red blood cells, and the red blood cells themselves are large and abnormally shaped. Vegan vegetarians are also more prone to develop B12 deficiency, because this nutrient is found primarily in animal protein, such as liver. Persons who have this deficiency must receive B12 injections in order to avoid the serious symptoms that can result. Vegans should consider taking a supplement of 2 mcg of B12 per day. Vitamin B12 deficiency can cause nervous system damage, mental disturbances, digestive symptoms, and slight yellowing of the skin.

Folic acid, another member of the vitamin B-complex, is also needed for the production of healthy red blood cells. Folic acid is an essential factor in the formation of heme, the iron-containing pigment found in hemoglobin.

As you recall, hemoglobin is the protein that carries oxygen in the red blood cells. Along with vitamin B12, it plays an important role in the breakdown and utilization of proteins. Like vitamin B12, a deficiency in folic acid hinders normal red blood cell production and creates large, abnormally shaped cells. Folic acid is also essential for healthy brain and nervous system function. Symptoms of folic acid deficiency include fatigue, depression, headaches, diarrhea, abdominal pain, soreness of the tongue, and cracking at the corners of the mouth. Folic acid deficiencies are common in women, especially teenagers and elderly women, because of poor nutritional habits. Alcoholics are at particular risk of developing folic acid deficiency.

The need for folic acid increases significantly during pregnancy for normal neural tube development in the fetus. (Low blood levels of folic acid are found in 20 percent of pregnant women.) Folic acid is found primarily in leafy green vegetables, soybeans and other legumes, and in liver—foods which do not figure significantly on the mainstream American menu. Folic acid is found primarily in leafy green vegetables and liver, which do not figure significantly in many women's diets. Also, women who use birth control pills for contraception or to regulate their cycles are at higher risk of developing folic acid deficiency.

Pyridoxine, or vitamin B6, is also necessary for normal red blood cell production. According to medical studies, anemia that fails to respond to iron may be corrected with daily supplements of vitamin B6. Other research suggests that patients with sickle-cell anemia have abnormally low levels of vitamin B6 in their red blood cells, levels that may be raised by supplementation.

Though iron, vitamin B12, folic acid, vitamin B6, and many other nutrients are necessary for red blood cell production, vitamin E is important for red blood cell survival. Medical research done on subjects deficient in vitamin E has shown that this nutrient helps to prolong the life span of red blood cells. Vitamin E also seems to help extend the life of the red blood cells in patients with cystic fibrosis and other types of pancreatic disease.

Women Are at Risk of Anemia Throughout Their Lives

Contraceptive Users: Intrauterine Devices, Birth Control Pills
Teenagers
Athletic Women in Training
Menstruating Women
Pregnant Women
Nursing Mothers
Elderly Women

Anemia is a problem that can complicate pre-existing health conditions. For example, anemia often accompanies rheumatoid arthritis, thyroid disease, and chronic kidney disease, as well as infections that tend to recur and become chronic. Anemia contributes to the fatigue and lack of energy that affect people suffering from these health problems.

Some anemias are genetically linked and are more prevalent in certain ethnic groups. Sickle-cell anemia is found in people of African descent and can cause severe symptoms, including episodes of fever and pain in the arms, legs, and abdomen. These symptoms can start in early childhood and are due to a decrease in the fluidity of the whole blood, which causes a blood flow obstruction in the small blood vessels. Another type of genetically linked anemia is thalassemia, which is found primarily in people of Southeast Asian or Mediterranean heritage. In severe cases, thalassemia causes an enlarged liver and spleen, as well as a very low red blood cell count. Infant mortality among those severely affected is quite high.

Anemia can be caused by drugs that destroy or interfere with utilization of the nutrients necessary for the health and maturation of the red blood cells. These drugs include oral contraceptives, alcohol, and anti-convulsive agents such as Dilantin. Exposure to radiation or to toxic chemicals, such as certain insecticides, may also damage the bone marrow, resulting in anemia.

Causes of Anemia

Nutritional Deficiencies
Minerals:
    Iron, copper, zinc
Vitamins:
    A; B-complex, especially folic
    acid, B12, B6; C; and E

Blood Loss
Excessive menstrual bleeding
Use of anti-inflammatory drugs
Intrauterine devices

Environmental Toxicity
Toxic chemical exposure
Radiation poisoning
Drug intake

Disease-Related Anemia
Thyroid disease
Rheumatoid arthritis
Kidney disease
Chronic infections
Malabsorption syndrome
Other chronic diseases

Part II:
Evaluating Your Symptoms

2

The Anemia Workbook

This workbook section will help you evaluate your symptoms as well as the factors that contribute to your risk of developing anemia. It is important to be aware of your risk factors since these problems can recur throughout your reproductive years and, in the case of anemia, well into your postmenopausal years. Fortunately, you can eliminate many risk factors by modifying your lifestyle habits.

If you take the time to fill out the evaluation sheets, you'll find it easier to recognize your weak areas; then you can put together your own treatment program from the following chapters for the best relief and prevention of anemia.

First, fill out the checklist to evaluate your symptoms. Then, carefully assess your responses for the risk factors for anemia. Finally, fill out the lifestyle habit evaluations related to eating and exercise. These will help you assess specific areas of your life to see which of your habit patterns are contributing to your symptoms. This evaluation will also show you if you are at risk for anemia. Working with the preventive health care techniques in the rest of the book can help improve your health and lessen your risks.

When you have completed the evaluations, you will be ready to go on to the next chapter and begin your treatment program.

Symptoms of Anemia

The most common symptoms of anemia are listed below. The first four symptoms may occur in women with heavy menstrual bleeding. Check the ones that pertain to you. Some women have very few symptoms, while others have symptoms severe enough to affect their ability to function normally. The worse your symptoms, the more important it is that you follow the self-help guidelines in this book.

	Yes	No
Abdominal pain	____	____
Dizziness	____	____
Fatigue	____	____
General weakness	____	____
Brittle nails	____	____
Paleness	____	____
Diarrhea	____	____
Loss of appetite	____	____
Sore tongue	____	____
Yellowing of skin	____	____
Tingling in hands and feet	____	____
Loss of coordination	____	____
Profuse or extended menstrual bleeding	____	____

Risk Factors for Anemia

You may have a higher likelihood of developing anemia if any of the following risk factors are positive. Women are especially vulnerable to developing anemia at certain times in their lives, such as adolescence, pregnancy, and premenopause. During these phases of your life, careful attention to prevention may be helpful. Risk factors linked to lifestyle issues, such as poor diet and nutrient intake, can be easily modified; see the nutritional section of this book.

	Yes	No
High dairy-product diet	___	___
Poor nutritional habits (high level of junk-food intake)	___	___
High wheat diet	___	___
Malabsorption syndrome, celiac disease, or sprue	___	___
Teenager	___	___
Heavy menstruation	___	___
Pregnancy	___	___
Peptic ulcer	___	___
Chronic use of laxatives	___	___
Chronic diarrhea	___	___
Dietary lack of folic acid, vitamin B12, other B-complex vitamins, vitamins A, C, and E, copper, and zinc from either food or supplements	___	___
Vegetarian without dietary or supplemental source of vitamin B12	___	___

Lifestyle Habits for Anemia

Eating Habits Checklist

Check the number of times you eat the following foods

Foods That Increase Symptoms

Foods	Never	1x a Month	1x a Week	>1x a Week
Coffee				
Cow's milk				
Cow's cheese				
Butter				
Chocolate				
Sugar				
Alcohol				
White bread				
Pasta				
Wheat bread				
Wheat noodles				
Wheat-based flour				
Pastries				
Added salt				
Bouillon				
Commercial salad dressing				
Catsup				
Black tea				
Soft drinks				
Hot dogs				
Ham				
Bacon				
Beef				
Lamb				
Pork				

Foods That Decrease Symptoms

Foods	Never	1x a Month	1x a Week	>1x a Week
Avocado				
Green Beans				
Beets				
Broccoli				
Brussels sprouts				
Cabbage				
Carrots				
Celery				
Collard greens				
Cucumbers				
Eggplant				
Garlic				
Horseradish				
Kale				
Legumes				
Lettuce				
Mustard greens				
Okra				
Onions				
Parsnips				
Peas				
Potatoes				
Radishes				
Rutabagas				
Spinach				
Squash				
Sweet potatoes				
Tomatoes				
Turnips				
Turnip greens				
Yams				
Brown rice				
Millet				
Barley				
Oatmeal				
Buckwheat				
Rye				
Raw flaxseeds				
Corn				

Raw pumpkin seeds				
Raw sesame seeds				
Raw sunflower seeds				
Raw almonds				
Raw filberts				
Raw pecans				
Raw walnuts				
Apples				
Bananas				
Berries				
Pears				
Seasonal fruits				
Corn oil				
Flax oil				
Olive oil				
Sesame oil				
Safflower oil				
Eggs				
Poultry				
Fish				

Key to Eating Habits

Anemia tendencies are greatly affected by the quality of your nutritional habits: The production of healthy red blood cells and the ability to regulate menstrual flow depend on an abundance of nutrients such as iron, vitamin B12, folic acid, vitamin B6, vitamin E, bioflavonoids, and vitamin C, as well as other essential nutrients.

All foods on the preceding list from avocados to poultry are high-nutrient, low-stress foods. Many contain one or more of the essential nutrients needed to relieve and prevent anemia. All foods from coffee to salami are high-stress foods that can worsen your anemia and menstrual bleeding problems. These are foods that are either low in essential nutrients needed for red blood cell formation or are risk factors for estrogen dominant related conditions like fibroid tumors and endometriosis that can promote heavy and irregular bleeding and create a higher risk of anemia as a result.

If you eat large numbers of these foods, or if you eat any of these foods frequently, your nutritional habits may be contributing significantly to your symptoms, and you can probably benefit greatly from the dietary guidelines in the nutritional chapters. In fact, hard-to-digest foods such as wheat and dairy products may even make your anemia worse. This is because they can have a detrimental effect on absorption and assimilation of essential nutrients, such as iron, that are needed for the production of healthy red blood cells.

Exercise Habits Checklist

Check the number of times you do each of the following activities:

Activity	Never	Once a Month	Once a Week	>Once a Week
Walking				
Swimming				
Bicycling				
Stretching				
Golf				
Weight lifting (low stress)				
T'ai chi				
Ballroom dancing				

Key to Exercise Habits

Many women with anemia tend to have major problems with fatigue as well as lack of physical endurance and stamina. Even women who have been used to an active and vigorous exercise regimen may feel that any physical activity at all is just too difficult and may decide to stop exercising completely. This can have negative physiological effects on the body and increase the symptoms. While vigorous exercise may indeed exhaust a woman suffering from anemia, gentle and moderate exercise can provide the benefits of oxygenation and improved blood circulation. Select one or two of the less strenuous exercises given in the checklist and do them two to three times per week.

Part III:
Finding the Solution

3

Vitamins, Minerals & Herbs

The use of vitamins, minerals, and herbs is extremely important for both the treatment and the prevention of anemia. In order to be symptom-free, you must have an optimal intake of the nutrients necessary for the growth and production of red blood cells and for the regulation of bleeding problems. Women with estrogen dominant related health issues like fibroid tumors, endometriosis and endometrial hyperplasia and pregnant women are at higher risk of developing anemia. Some women become anemic through intestinal or other blood loss. I have found that my patients heal most effectively when they combine the right mix of nutritional supplements with a nutrient-rich diet.

In order to restore the level of nutrients necessary to produce an adequate number of red blood cells as well as healthy red blood cells, dietary intake alone is often not sufficient. Anemic women often need to both take nutritional supplements and follow a healthy diet to "jump start" the system into healthy blood production as well as reduce blood loss because of heavy and irregular menstrual or intestinal bleeding. Nutritional supplements can help reestablish a healthy hormonal profile, as well as restore the strength and integrity of the capillaries and other blood vessels so that normal bleeding patterns resume.

As you read this chapter, you will also learn about the beneficial effects that nutritional supplements can have in treating the fatigue, depression, low energy, poor digestion, and other symptoms of anemia. In fact, poor or inadequate nutrition may play a major role in causing these problems or contribute greatly to their onset.

This chapter is divided into three sections. The first discusses the role of vitamins and minerals in the body, along with their major food sources. The next section discusses which herbs are helpful for anemia and why they are effective. The third section gives specific recommendations on how to use these supplements. A sample nutritional supplement formula for anemia is included. Towards the end of the chapter, I have included several charts listing major food sources of each essential nutrient. The importance of nutrition in regulating anemia is supported by numerous medical studies done at university centers and hospitals.

Vitamins and Minerals for Anemia

Vitamin A: Vitamin A is necessary for the normal growth and support of the eyes, skin, and mucous membranes and healthy immune function. Deficiency of vitamin A results in impaired immune function, rough, scaly skin, and night blindness. It is also needed for the healthy production of red blood cells. In an interesting study of middle-aged men on a diet deficient in vitamin A, it was found that the hemoglobin count started to decline even before a change in night vision or a measurable deficiency in the vitamin A levels was noted. In a study of 71 women with excessive bleeding, the women were found to have significantly lower blood levels of vitamin A than the normal population. Almost 90 percent of the women studied returned to a normal bleeding pattern after two weeks of vitamin A treatment.

There are two types of vitamin A. Vitamin A from animal sources usually comes from fish liver and is oil soluble. This type of vitamin A can be toxic if taken in too large a dose (i.e., greater than 25,000 international units [I.U.] per day, if taken for more than a few months). In contrast, beta carotene, the precursor of vitamin A found in plants, is water soluble and is not toxic in large amounts. A single sweet potato or cup of carrot juice contains more than 20,000 I.U. of beta carotene.

Vitamin B-Complex: The vitamin B-complex consists of eleven factors that work together to perform many important biochemical functions in the body. These functions include stabilization of brain chemistry, glucose metabolism, and the inactivation of estrogen by the liver. Since heavy menstrual bleeding can be due to excess estrogen in the body, it is important that estrogen levels are properly regulated through breakdown and disposal by the liver. Vitamin B factors are essential for healthy liver functioning.

The B-complex vitamins are also necessary for the prevention and reversal of anemia. A deficiency of vitamin B1 (thiamine), vitamin B2 (riboflavin), vitamin B5 (pantothenic acid), and vitamin B6 (pyridoxine) may cause anemia, even in people who have no deficiencies in iron, folic acid, or vitamin B12. The B-complex vitamins are commonly found in foods such as whole grains, beans and peas, and liver. These vitamins are water soluble. When a woman is under emotional stress, the B-complex vitamins are more easily lost from the body. This can worsen the fatigue and lack of vitality from which women with anemia already suffer. Dosage is 25 to 100 mg per day.

Folic Acid: Folic acid is one of the B-complex vitamins and is an important nutrient for women. It helps prevent cervical dysplasia, a condition that can be a precursor to cancer of the cervix. It is also a necessary supplement for women who use birth control pills, since oral contraceptives interfere with folic acid absorption. Deficiency of folic acid in pregnant women has been linked to neural tube defects in their babies, such as spina bifida. Folic acid plays an important role in the production of red blood cells.

A deficiency of folic acid leads to anemia that cannot be corrected by supplemental iron. With folic acid deficiency, red blood cells don't mature properly; they are large and irregularly shaped. Drugs that interfere with proper folic acid absorption include sulfa drugs and other antibiotics, alcohol, phenobarbital, and anticonvulsants used in the treatment of epilepsy. Women with folic acid deficiency anemia are prone to symptoms such as sore tongue, digestive disturbances, forgetfulness, and mental confusion. Good food sources of folic acid include oysters, salmon, whole grains, and green leafy vegetables. Dosage is 400 mg to 1 gram per day.

Vitamin B12: Vitamin B12 is a water-soluble vitamin that plays an important role in the production of red blood cells. Like a deficiency in folic acid, a B12 deficiency causes retardation in the growth and development of the red blood cells. Vitamin B12 is poorly absorbed from the gastro-intestinal tract if the intrinsic factor, a necessary enzyme, is deficient. Since vitamin B12 is found primarily in meat, vegetarians may be at risk of developing a B12 deficiency.

Symptoms of this deficiency develop slowly and may not become apparent for as long as five or six years. A deficiency of B12 causes symptoms such as shooting pains, pins-and-needles or hot-and-cold sensations in the extremities, as well as numbness, stiffness, and difficulty in walking. It can also cause mental disturbances similar to psychosis, as well as memory defects and mental slowness. In order to treat B12 deficiency anemia (or pernicious anemia), the digestive tract must be bypassed and the B12 given as injections.

Vitamin C: This important anti-stress vitamin is necessary for proper adrenal function as well as for immune function. Vitamin C increases iron absorption from the non-heme iron sources such as bran, peas, seeds, nuts, and leafy green vegetables. This can help to prevent iron deficiency anemia. Vitamin C has also been tested, along with bioflavonoids, as a treatment for heavy menstrual bleeding.

One study showed a reduction in bleeding in 87 percent of the women participating. Vitamin C strengthens capillaries and prevents capillary fragility, which can lead to excessive bleeding. Fruits and vegetables are excellent sources of vitamin C. Dosage is 800 to 2000 mg per day.

Soy Isoflavones: Genistein and diadzein are isoflavones found in soy with weak estrogen-like activity. They help to reduce excess estrogen levels by interfering with estrogen production and the binding of estrogen to tissues such as the breast and uterus. In fact, a study of Hawaiian women found that using soy actively reduced the risk of endometrial (uterine) cancer by 54 percent.

Bioflavonoids: Bioflavonoids have chemical activity similar to estrogen and can be used as an estrogen substitute. Interestingly, bioflavonoids contain a very low potency of estrogen, much lower than that produced in our own bodies. When you take bioflavonoids supplements, they bind to hormone receptor sites that affect the conversion of testosterone to estrogen by the ovaries and adrenal glands, thereby lowering your own production of potent estrogen and substituting a weaker plant source of this hormone. This can be helpful in the treatment of estrogen dominance that is a very common cause of heavy menstrual bleeding and anemia. Bioflavonoids are very safe to use and side effects are minimal and infrequent.

Bioflavonoids, along with vitamin C, also reduce heavy menstrual bleeding due to hormonal imbalance by strengthening the capillary walls. They have even been used to treat women who have lost multiple pregnancies due to bleeding. In nature, bioflavonoids are found in fruits, such as citrus rind and pulp, grape skins, cherries, blackberries, as well as vegetables. Dosage is 700 to 2000 mg per day.

Flaxseeds: Flaxseeds contain both omega-3 essential fatty acids and lignans which make up the cellular wall of the seeds. Both substances are weakly estrogenic and help to reduce estrogen levels within the body, as well as promoting healthy ovulation which is necessary for the production of progesterone during the second half of the menstrual cycle. Progesterone helps to limit heavy menstrual bleeding so helps to eliminate a major cause of anemia. This was researched with positive results in a study on flaxseed promoting more regular ovulation done at the University of Michigan. In my medical practice I have found flaxseed oil to be an effective menstrual regulator. Use 1 to 3 tablespoons per day as an oil or butter substitute.

Vitamin E: Vitamin E can act as a weak estrogen substitute. It has been studied as a treatment for hot flashes, the psychological symptoms of menopause, and even vaginal dryness. In one study, vitamin E was found to help skew the estrogen-progesterone ratio in the body toward progesterone and is needed for normal ovulation. It is helpful for those women who have heavy menstrual bleeding due to excess estrogen. Vitamin E also protects the cells from the destructive effects of environmental pollutants that can react with the cell membrane. It increases red blood cell survival and is an important nutrient for the prevention of anemia. Vitamin E is found in wheat germ, nuts, and seeds. Dosage is 400 to 1600 IU per day.

Iron: Women who suffer from heavy menstrual bleeding tend to be iron deficient. In fact, some medical studies have found that inadequate iron intake may be a cause of excessive bleeding as well as an effect of the problem. Women who suffer from heavy menstrual bleeding should have their red blood count checked to see if supplemental iron is necessary, in addition to adopting a high-iron-content diet. Heme iron, the iron from meat sources such as liver, is much better absorbed and assimilated than non-heme iron, the iron from vegetarian sources. To be absorbed properly, non-heme iron must be taken with at least 75 milligrams of vitamin C. For more information about food combinations that are high in both iron and vitamin C, see the following two chapters on dietary planning.

Iron deficiency is the main cause of anemia. Iron is an essential component of red blood cells, combining with protein and copper to make hemoglobin, the pigment of the red blood cells. Iron deficiency is common during all phases of a woman's life and is a frequent cause of fatigue and low-energy states. Good food sources of iron include liver, blackstrap molasses, beans and peas, seeds and nuts, and certain fruits and vegetables.

Copper: Copper aids in the formation of red blood cells. A deficiency of copper is associated with anemia, since copper is necessary for proper iron absorption. Copper is found in all body tissues and is present in many of the enzymes that break down and build up body tissues. The best food sources of copper include liver, whole grains, legumes, seafood, and green leafy vegetables.

Zinc: Zinc plays an important role in the body. It is a constituent of many enzymes involved both in metabolism and digestion. It is also needed for the proper growth and development of female reproductive organs and for the normal functioning of the male prostate gland. Good food sources of zinc include wheat germ, pumpkin seeds, whole grains, wheat bran, and high-protein foods. Persons who have sickle-cell anemia may be deficient in zinc. One interesting clinical study showed a decrease in the number of sick-led red blood cells in patients who used zinc supplementation.

Nutrients	Importance
Vitamins	
Vitamin A	Deficiency is associated with anemia due to impaired hemoglobin synthesis as well as heavy menstrual bleeding.
Vitamin B_1 (thiamine)	Deficiency may cause megaloblastic (large-shaped cells) anemia.
Vitamin B_2 (riboflavin)	Aids in formation of red blood cells. Deficiency is associated with anemia.
Vitamin B_5 (pantothenic acid)	Aids in the reversal of anemia in cases with increased iron storage in the bone marrow.
Vitamin B_6 (pyridoxine)	Deficiency causes anemia.
Vitamin B_{12} (cyanocobalamin)	Essential for normal formation of blood cells and prevention of pernicious anemia.
Folic Acid (folacin)	Necessary for red blood cell formation.
Vitamin C	Aids in absorption of iron. Deficiency is associated with heavy menstrual bleeding.
Soy Isoflavones	Helps to reduce excess estrogen.
Bioflavonoids	Deficiency is associated with heavy menstrual bleeding.
Flaxseed Oil	Promotes healthy ovulation.
Vitamin E	Protects red blood cells from destruction. Important for sickle-cell anemia and anemia associated with cystic fibrosis and pancreatic insufficiency.
Minerals	
Copper	Aids in formation of red blood cells. Deficiency is associated with anemia.
Nutrients	Importance
Iron	Necessary for hemoglobin formation. Deficiency causes most frequent type of anemia.
Zinc	May be deficient in sickle-cell anemia.
Other Factors	
Hydrochloric acid	If deficient, may affect iron deficiency anemia.

Herbs for Anemia

Herbs can play a helpful role in your nutritional program to relieve and prevent anemia. They should be thought of as a form of extended nutrition that can be taken as either teas or capsules. Two herbs have been traditionally used to stop excessive menstrual flow and postpartum hemorrhage: golden seal and shepherd's purse. Recent research studies have supported the traditional claims made for these herbs. Golden seal contains a chemical called berberine that calms uterine muscular tension. It has also been used to calm and soothe the digestive tract.

Shepherd's purse helps promote blood clotting and has also been used to help stop menstrual bleeding. If your bleeding is excessive or irregular, consult your physician. This needs to be evaluated carefully by your physician and, if necessary, medical therapy should be instituted. Excessive and irregular bleeding can be dangerous and should never be allowed to continue without medical help. For those women for whom the menstrual flow is normal but somewhat heavier than usual, the mild properties of herbs may be helpful for symptom relief.

Plants that contain bioflavonoids may also help stop and prevent heavy menstrual bleeding. Bioflavonoids help to strengthen capillaries and, along with vitamin C, can help prevent excessive bruising as well as bleeding. They are found in the rind and pulp of citrus fruits, hawthorn berries, bilberries, cherries, and grape skins. Other herbs help to prevent anemia by providing good sources of non-heme iron. Excellent examples are yellow dock and pau d'arco. Other plants help to relieve heavy menstrual bleeding by reducing elevated levels of estrogen in the body. Soy and red clover contain estrogen-like isoflavones which both interfere with estrogen production and block the estrogen from binding to breast and uterine tissues.

Plants that improve the detoxification and breakdown of estrogen by the liver also help to reduce excessive amounts of estrogen within the body. One such herb is tumeric, or curcumin (its active ingredient), which is a traditional flavoring in Indian food.

Vitex agnus, or chasteberry, has been found to improve the estrogen-to-progesterone ratio in the body by favoring the production of progesterone during the second half of the menstrual cycle. This helps limit the amount of blood lost with menstruation. Vitex acts by promoting ovulation at mid-cycle through stimulating the production of the pituitary luteinizing hormone (LK).

Silymarin, or milk thistle, protects liver functions through its flavonoid content. These flavonoids are strong antioxidants and help protect the liver from damage.

How to Use Vitamin, Mineral & Herbal Supplements

Good dietary habits and the use of nutritional supplements are a necessary combination for women who want to make up the nutritional deficiencies that accompany anemia. In order to restore the level of nutrients necessary to produce an adequate number of red blood cells as well as healthy red blood cells, dietary intake may not be sufficient. Anemic women may need to take nutritional supplements and follow a healthy diet to "jump start" the system into normal functioning again. This is also true for women with heavy menstrual bleeding; nutritional supplements can help reestablish a healthy hormonal profile, as well as restore the strength and integrity of the capillaries and other blood vessels so that normal bleeding patterns resume.

Vitamin, mineral, and herbal supplements, however, should never be used as an excuse to continue poor dietary habits. They should be taken only with high-nutrient meals to maintain optimal health. With anemia, it is important to make sure that both your diet and your supplement program provide the extra nutrients that your body needs.

On the following page is a sample nutritional supplement formula to support healthy blood formation as well as hormonal health. I do want to emphasize, however, that any anemia problem should be evaluated by a physician. Nutritional support should not be used to replace medical therapy when anima occurs.

Remember that all women differ somewhat in their nutritional needs. If you do take the recommended supplements for either problem, I usually recommend that you start with one-fourth to one-half of the dose recommended in this book, then slowly work your way up to a higher dosage. You may find that you feel best with slightly more or less of certain ingredients.

I recommend that all supplements be taken with meals or at least with a snack. A digestive reaction to supplements, such as nausea or indigestion, is rare. If this happens to you, stop all supplements and start them again one at a time until you find the offending nutrient. Any nutrient to which you have a reaction should be eliminated from your program. If you have any specific questions, ask a healthcare professional who is knowledgeable about nutrition.

Summary Chart For Nutritional Supplements

I want to end this section by summarizing the nutritional supplements that you can take to help eliminate your anemia symptoms. These include:

1. **Vitamins and Minerals** - Vitamin A, Vitamin B-Complex, Folic Acid, Vitamin B12, Vitamin C, Soy Isoflavones, Bioflavonoids, Flaxseeds, Vitamin E, Iron, Copper, Zinc.

2. **Herbs** – golden seal, shepherd's purse, yellow dock, pau d'arco, red clover, turmeric, vitex agnus (chasteberry) and silymarin (milk thistle).

Optimal Nutritional Supplementation for Anemia

Vitamins and Minerals	Maximum Daily Dose
Vitamin A	5000 I.U.
Beta-carotene (provitamin A)	10,000 – 25,000 I.U.
Vitamin B-Complex	
B1 (thiamine)	25 - 100 mg
B2 (riboflavin)	25 - 100 mg
B3 (niacinamide)	25 - 100 mg
B5 (pantothenic acid)	25 - 100 mg
B6 (pyridoxine)	50 – 100 mg
B12 (cyanocobalamin)	100 – 750 mcg
Folic acid	400 – 800 mcg
Biotin	200 - 500 mcg
Choline	25 - 100 mg
Inositol	25 - 100 mg
PABA	25 - 100 mg
Vitamin C	1000-4000 mg
(as mineral ascorbates)	
Vitamin D	1000 I.U.
Bioflavonoids	1000-2000 mg
Rutin	200 mg
Vitamin E	800-1600 I.U.
(d-alpha tocopherol acetate)	
Calcium	1000 - 1200 mg
Magnesium	500 - 600 mg
Potassium	100 mg
Iron	18 -25 mg (for maintenance)
	30-60 mg (for treatment)
Zinc	15 mg
Iodine	150 mcg
Manganese	5 mg
Copper	2 mg
Selenium	200 mcg
Chromium	100 – 200 mcg
Boron	3 mg

Food Sources of Iron

Grains
Bran cereal
Millet, dry
Wheat germ
Pasta, whole wheat
Bran muffin
Pumpernickel bread
Oak flakes
Shredded wheat
Whole wheat bread
Rye bread
Wheat bran
Pearl barley
White rice

Legumes
Black beans
Pinto beans
Garbanzo beans
Soybeans
Kidney beans
Lima beans
Lentils
Split peas
Black-eyed peas
Green peas
Tofu

Vegetables
Brussels sprouts
Spinach
Broccoli
Sweet potatoes
Dandelion greens
Green beans
Corn
Leeks
Kale
Swiss chard
Beets
Beet greens
Mushrooms
Parsnips
Carrots
Mustard greens
Green pepper
Lettuce
Turnips
Asparagus
Collards
Cauliflower
Zucchini
Winter squash
Red cabbage

More Food Sources of Iron

Fruits	Meat, Poultry, Seafood	Nuts and Seeds
Prune juice	Calf's liver	Sesame seeds
Figs	Beef liver	Sunflower seeds
Raisins	Chicken liver	Pistachios
Prunes, dried	Oysters	Pecans
Avocado	Trout	Sesame butter
Apple juice	Clams	Almonds
Dates, dried	Scallops	Hazelnuts (filberts)
Blackberries	Sardines	Walnuts
Pineapple	Shrimp	
Grape juice	Chicken	
Apricots, fresh	Haddock	
Cantaloupe	Cod	
Strawberries	Salmon	
Cherries		

Food Sources of Vitamin A

Fruits	Meat, Poultry, Seafood	Vegetables
Apricots	Crab	Carrots
Avocado	Halibut	Carrot juice
Cantaloupe	Liver*—all types	Collard greens
Mangoes	Mackerel	Dandelion greens
Papaya	Salmon	Green onions
Peaches	Swordfish	Kale
Persimmons		Parsley
		Spinach
		Sweet potatoes
		Turnip greens
		Winter squash

Eggs and meat must be from range fed, organic sources fed on non-pesticide fodder.

Food Sources of Vitamin B-Complex
(including folic acid)

Vegetables, Legumes
Alfalfa
Artichoke
Asparagus
Beets
Broccoli
Brussels sprouts
Cabbage
Cauliflower
Corn
Garbanzo beans
Green beans
Kale
Leeks
Lentils
Lima beans
Onions
Peas
Pinto beans
Romaine lettuce
Soybeans

Meat, Poultry, Seafood
Egg yolks
Liver*

Grains
Barley
Bran
Brown rice
Corn
Millet
Rice bran
Wheat
Wheat germ

Sweeteners
Blackstrap molasses

Food Sources of Vitamin B$_6$

Grains
Brown rice
Buckwheat flour
Rice bran
Rye flour
Wheat germ
Whole wheat flour

Meat, Poultry, Seafood
Seafood
Chicken
Salmon
Tuna

Vegetables
Asparagus
Beet greens
Broccoli
Brussels sprouts
Cauliflower
Green peas
Leeks
Sweet potatoes

Nuts and seeds
Sunflower
Seeds

Food sources for Vitamin B$_{12}$

Protein	Eggs
Fish	Liver

Food Sources of Vitamin C

Fruits	*Vegetables, Legumes*
Blackberries	Asparagus
Black currants	Black-eyed peas
Cantaloupe	Broccoli
Elderberries	Brussels sprouts
Grapefruit	Cabbage
Grapefruit juice	Cauliflower
Guavas	Collards
Kiwi fruit	Green onions
Mangoes	Green peas
Oranges	Kale
Orange juice	Kohlrabi
Pineapple	Parsley
Raspberries	Potatoes
Strawberries	Rutabaga
Tangerines	Sweet peppers
	Sweet potatoes
Meat, Poultry, Seafood	Tomatoes
Liver – all types	Turnips
Pheasant	
Quail	
Salmon	

Food Sources of Copper

Vegetables, Legumes
Kidney beans
Lentils
Lima beans
Okra
Split peas

Meat, Poultry, Seafood
Liver
Cod
Haddock
Halibut
Lobster
Oysters
Pike
Shrimp

Fruits
Avocado
Dried figs
Prunes
Raisins

Nuts and seeds
Almonds
Filberts
Pecans
Pistachios
Sesame seeds
Sunflower seeds
Walnuts

Sweeteners
Blackstrap
molasses

Food Sources of Zinc

Grains
Barley
Brown rice
Buckwheat
Corn
Cornmeal
Millet
Oatmeal
Rice bran
Rye bread
Wheat bran
Wheat germ
Wheat berries
Whole wheat bread
Whole wheat flour

Vegetables, Legumes
Black-eyed peas
Cabbage
Carrots
Garbanzo beans
Green peas
Lentils
Lettuce
Lima beans
Onions
Soy flour
Soy meal
Soy

Meat, Poultry, Seafood
Chicken
Oysters

Fruits
Apples
Peaches

4

Menus, Meal Plans & Recipes

Many of my patients with anemia have asked me for specific recipes and meal plans to help optimize their healing program. Unfortunately, many cookbooks have dishes that look and taste great but are laden with ingredients that can actually worsen a woman's health issues—including high-stress foods such as dairy products, unhealthy saturated fats, chocolate, sugar, and caffeinated beverages. Some cookbooks do present low-calorie "light dishes." Although these cookbooks eliminate unhealthy fats and sugars from the recipes, they still don't give a woman with anemia the therapeutic levels of specific nutrients she needs.

To answer this need, I have developed a number of meal plans and recipes specifically for women. These recipes not only provide essential nutrients for healthy blood formation but will also help restore hormonal health and combat estrogen dominance. Women's health issues like fibroid tumors and endometriosis are related to estrogen dominance. They often cause the heavy menstrual bleeding that leads to anemia.

Not only have the recipes been designed to look and taste good, but they contain high levels of the nutrients you need to help rebuild and repair your body as well as those needed to help prevent anemia.

However, no one diet fits the needs of all different body types. Because of this I have included menus and delicious recipes for women who prefer a vegetarian emphasis, high complex carbohydrate diet as well as dishes and entrees for women who feel their best on a high protein, meat-based diet. All of these meal plans and the recipes in the next chapter contain ingredients that are very beneficial for women who are dealing with issues related to PMS as well as other health issues. In addition, the high stress ingredients that can worsen your symptoms have been eliminated

The recipes I have included in this chapter are quick and easy to prepare. Most women have very busy lives, and I have found that anything too complicated won't work for me or my patients. Best of all, these recipes are delicious and satisfying as well as healthful. I hope that you enjoy them as much as I do.

Breakfast Menus

These delicious, easy to prepare menus will provide a variety of healthful and delicious meals. They can also act as guidelines as you create your own meal plans. I have developed them for their content of the essential nutrients that help to build healthy red blood cells.

Flax shake with protein powder
and fresh fruit
~~~~~~~~~~~~~~~

Blueberry and spirulina smoothie
~~~~~~~~~~~~~~~

Millet cereal with raisins and
cinnamon
Nondairy yogurt
Chamomile tea
~~~~~~~~~~~~~~~

Rice and flaxseed pancakes
Banana
Vanilla nondairy milk
~~~~~~~~~~~~~~~

Oatmeal with raspberries
Chamomile tea
~~~~~~~~~~~~~~~

Nondairy yogurt with granola
and ground flaxseed
Peppermint tea
~~~~~~~~~~~~~~~

Scrambled eggs with turkey
bacon
Lemon ginger tea
Orange slices
~~~~~~~~~~~~~~~

Omelette with chicken sausage
Roasted grain beverage
(coffee substitute)
Apple slices
~~~~~~~~~~~~~~~

Lunch and Dinner Menus

These scrumptious menus give you a variety of ways to organize your meals. Use them as guidelines to design your own meal plans. All these dishes were chosen because they contain many nutrients helpful for anemia.

Soup Meals

Split pea soup
Corn muffins
Fresh applesauce
~~~~~~~~~~~~~~

Chicken and wild rice soup
Cole slaw
Millet bread with flax oil
~~~~~~~~~~~~~~

Vegetable soup with brown rice
Steamed kale
Baked potato with flax oil
Apple slices
~~~~~~~~~~~~~~

Lentil soup
Herbed brown rice
Broccoli with lemon
~~~~~~~~~~~~~~

Tomato soup
Potato salad with low-fat mayonnaise
Celery and carrot sticks
~~~~~~~~~~~~~~

Salad Meals

Spinach salad with turkey bacon or tofu
Corn muffins with flax oil
Orange slices
~~~~~~~~~~~~~~

Beet salad with goat cheese
Rice crackers with fresh fruit preserves
~~~~~~~~~~~~~~

Romaine salad with grilled salmon and vinaigrette dressing
Gluten-free bread and olive oil dip
~~~~~~~~~~~~~~

Low-fat potato salad
Cole slaw
Hard boiled eggs
Melon slices
~~~~~~~~~~~~~~

Mixed Vegetable Salad with Kidney Beans
Baked yam

Meat Meals

Poached salmon with lemon
Herbed brown rice
Steamed carrots with honey
~~~~~~~~~~~~~

Roasted chicken with herbs
Baked potato with flax oil
Broccoli with lemon
~~~~~~~~~~~~~

Broiled trout with dill
Mixed green salad with vinaigrette
Green peas and onions
Apple slices
~~~~~~~~~~~~~

Grilled shrimp with olive oil and lemon
Wild rice
Steamed kale
~~~~~~~~~~~~~

One-Dish Vegetable Meals

Vegetarian tacos with black beans, brown rice, avocados, tomatoes, lettuce and low-salt salsa
~~~~~~~~~~~~~

Stir-fry with mixed vegetables, brown rice and tofu
Orange slices
~~~~~~~~~~~~~

Pasta with tomato sauce, broccoli, carrots, olive oil and garlic
Green salad with vinaigrette
~~~~~~~~~~~~~

Hummus dip
Eggplant dip (babaganoush)
Mixed raw vegetable slices including carrots, red bell peppers, and radishes
~~~~~~~~~~~~~

Brown rice and almond tabouli
Mixed olives
Melon slices
~~~~~~~~~~~~~

Note: Try to prepare your cooked dishes with an iron frying pan or skillet. Iron from the skillet will be absorbed by the food. This adds additional supplemental iron for those women with iron deficiency.

Breakfast Recipes

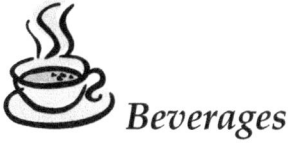 *Beverages*

These drinks are made with therapeutic herbal teas, power smoothies that are rich in fruits, raw seeds, nuts, protein powder, green foods and nondairy milk that are recommended for preventing and treating your symptoms.

The ingredients contain high levels of essential nutrients that help regulate your hormonal balance and help promote healthy blood formation. You can enjoy these beverages throughout the month, and not just during your symptom time if you are suffering from an estrogen dominant condition. The high mineral and other nutrient content in these drinks is beneficial for the entire body.

Relaxant Herb Tea   **Serves 2**

2 cups water
1 teaspoon chamomile leaves
1 teaspoon peppermint leaves
1 teaspoon honey (if desired)

Bring the water to a boil. Place herbs in water and stir. Turn heat to low and simmer for 15 minutes.

Peppermint and chamomile are both muscle relaxants and antispasmodic herbs, so they can provide relief of pain and cramping caused by fibroid tumors and endometriosis. They also help calm the mood.

Ginger Tea   **Serves 4**

Ginger makes a warming, delicious tea and is beneficial to your circulation. It is also a powerful anti-inflammatory herb. If the tea is too strong add more water.

5 cups water
3 tablespoons ginger coarsely chopped
½ lemon (optional)
Honey (or other sweetener, to taste)

Add ginger to the water in a cooking pot. Bring to a boil and then turn heat to low. Steep for 15 or 20 minutes. Squeeze lemon into tea and serve with honey or your favorite sweetener.

Blueberry Pomegranate Smoothie   **Serves 2**

¼ cup nondairy yogurt, unsweetened
¾ cup pomegranate juice
1 cup blueberries, fresh or frozen
1 tablespoon ground flaxseed
1 banana

Combine all ingredients in a blender. Puree until smooth and serve.

Raspberry Flax Smoothie   **Serves 2**

This creamy smoothie makes a great breakfast. Flaxseed oil one is my favorite foods. It is both delicious and rich in healthy omega-3 fatty acids. It also adds extra creaminess to the smoothie.

1 cup rice milk
⅔ cup raspberries – fresh or frozen
1 heaping tablespoon rice protein powder
1 tablespoon flaxseed oil
2 bananas, sliced

Combine all ingredients in a blender. Puree until smooth and serve.

Delicious Green Drink   Serves 1

½ cup Concord grape juice
¼ cup water
1 tablespoon ground flaxseed
½ teaspoon chlorella powder
½ teaspoon spirulina powder

Mix all ingredients together in a glass or puree in a blender.

Heavenly Strawberry Coconut Smoothie   Serves 2

This drink fits its name! It is absolutely scrumptious as well as good for you. If you don't have a high-speed blender and you are using whole raw cashews I recommend that you chop them up beforehand. Otherwise, raw cashew butter is a good substitute.

1 cup coconut drink, unsweetened (Coconut Dream brand preferred)
1 cup strawberries – fresh or frozen
1 tablespoon raw coconut flour
1 tablespoon raw cashews (about cashews 10-15)
1 banana, sliced

Combine all ingredients in a blender. Puree until smooth and serve.

Simple Flax Smoothie   Serves 2

Flaxseed is not only a tasty addition to smoothies but it is also very nutritious. Flaxseed is high in essential fatty acids, calcium, magnesium, and potassium.

1 cup vanilla nondairy milk
2 tablespoons ground flaxseed
1 banana

Combine all ingredients in a blender. Blend until smooth and serve.

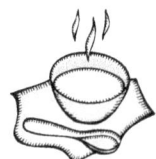 *Healthy, Quick Breakfasts*

Most American breakfasts include wheat and dairy products, such as yogurt, wheat toast, wheat cereal with milk, sweet rolls, and other wheat-based pastries. As I mentioned previously, dairy products and wheat can worsen the symptoms of estrogen dominant conditions like fibroid tumors and endometriosis that can be the cause of anemia by triggering heavy menstrual bleeding.

I have included in this section both whole grain, carbohydrate-based entrees as well as protein-rich dishes. Depending on the type of diet that makes you feel your best. Both types of entrees, however, will benefit estrogen dominance by eliminating wheat and dairy products at breakfast.

The whole grain dishes are based on ground flaxseed, soy, and gluten-free grains, all of which can be useful in reducing your symptoms. The protein-rich entrees have been created using eggs and healthy breakfast meats. Gluten, the protein found in wheat, can trigger symptoms of bloating, digestive disturbances, and fatigue.

Quinoa Cereal with Blueberries   **Serves 2**

1 ½ cups cooked quinoa
1 cup nondairy milk
½ cup blueberries
2 teaspoons honey or other sweetener

Combine quinoa and nondairy milk in a saucepan. Simmer for 5 minutes. Stir in honey and garnish with raspberries.

Quinoa with Prunes   **Serves 2**

This is one of my all-time favorite hot cereals. The plums are delicious and add a nice texture. Quinoa is a small, protein rich grain. When cooked the grains are small and fluffy. I recommend making a pot of quinoa the night before.

1 ½ cups cooked quinoa
1 cup nondairy milk
4-6 dried prunes, chopped
2 tablespoons flaxseed oil
2 teaspoons xylitol, honey, or maple syrup (if using unsweetened milk)
Pinch of salt (optional)

In a saucepan combine quinoa, nondairy milk, salt, and dried plums. Heat thoroughly and simmer on low heat for 5-10 minutes until plums have softened. Serve with flaxseed oil and sweetener.

Maple Cinnamon Oatmeal   **Serves 2**

1 cup gluten-free quick oats
1 ¾ cups water
1-2 tablespoons flaxseed oil
2 teaspoons maple syrup
Pinch of cinnamon (to taste)
Pinch of salt

Boil water in a saucepan. Add gluten-free oats and reduce to medium heat. Cook for one minute and stir. Cover, and remove oatmeal from heat. Serve in 2-3 minutes.

Stir in maple syrup, flaxseed oil, cinnamon and salt.

Strawberries and Cream Oatmeal **Serves 2**

1 cup gluten-free quick oats
½ cup strawberries, chopped
½ nondairy milk
1 ¼ cups water
1-2 tablespoons flaxseed oil
2 teaspoons honey or stevia
Pinch of salt (optional)

Bring water and nondairy milk to a boil in a saucepan. Add gluten-free oats and reduce to medium heat. Cook for one minute and stir. Cover, and remove oatmeal from heat. Serve in 2-3 minutes. Stir in sweetener, flaxseed oil, salt and top with strawberries.

Apple Almond Muffins **Makes 14-18**

The cinnamon and apples in these muffins makes the kitchen smell delicious and welcoming. If you are eating a nut-free diet simply omit the nuts.

2 cups rice flour
1 apple, diced (Granny Smith apple preferred)
½ cup applesauce
6 packets of Truvia (equal to ¼ cup sugar)
1 tablespoon honey
½ cup water
1 egg
3 tablespoons safflower oil
¼ cup chopped almonds
1 teaspoon cinnamon
¼ teaspoon nutmeg
1 teaspoon baking powder
½ teaspoon baking soda
Pinch of salt

Preheat oven to 400 degrees. Mix all dry ingredients and wet ingredients separately. Combine and pour a large spoonful (approximately a heaping tablespoon) into each muffin cup. I recommend using baking cups for this recipe. Bake for 20 minutes until cooked through.

Pumpkin Muffins **Makes 14-18**

1½ cups rice flour
½ teaspoon baking powder
½ teaspoon baking soda
1 cup pumpkin
1 teaspoon cinnamon
¼ teaspoon nutmeg
¼ cup chopped almonds (optional)
3 tablespoons molasses
3 tablespoons safflower oil
½ cup raisins
2 eggs
½ cup nondairy milk
1 teaspoon vanilla extract
Pinch of salt

Preheat oven to 400 degrees. Line a muffin tin with paper muffin cups. Combine all dry ingredients and mix thoroughly. In a separate bowl beat the two eggs and then combine the remainder of the wet ingredients. Add the wet ingredients to the dry and mix thoroughly.

Fill muffin cups ⅔ with the batter. Cook for 18-20 minutes or until thoroughly cooked.

Flaxseed Pancakes   **Makes 8 pancakes (Serves 2-4)**

Xylitol is an excellent sugar substitute for cooking and baking that can be found at most health food stores. Xylitol is easy to use because it has a 1:1 ratio with sugar. Yet, this product has 40% fewer calories than sugar and is beneficial for your teeth and gums.

1 cup gluten-free flour
1 cup unsweetened rice milk
1 egg
2 tablespoons xylitol
1 tablespoon ground flaxseed
1 teaspoon baking powder
½ teaspoon baking soda
¼ teaspoon salt
3 tablespoons almond oil, keeping 1 tbsp. for cooking
Maple syrup (optional)
Fruit jam (optional)

Mix the dry and wet ingredients in separate bowls. Combine all the ingredients and mix thoroughly. Cook on medium heat and use a small amount of oil to grease the pan if needed. When pancakes bubble in the center flip and cook for 1-2 minutes until cooked thoroughly. Serve with maple syrup or all-fruit jam. Delicious!

Egg and Sausage Scramble   **Serves 2**

4 eggs
4 turkey breakfast sausages
2 slice of gluten-free toast
Salt and pepper (optional)
2 teaspoons olive oil
Serve with ½ cup applesauce

Warm a frying pan on medium heat and add olive oil. Beat egg gently in a small bowl and set aside. Chop the sausages into small pieces - this will help them to cook faster. Add sausages to the pan and cook for several minutes until sausages are brown.

Turn heat to low and add eggs to the pan and scramble with the sausage. Add a pinch of salt and pepper. Serve with toast and applesauce. Bake for 20-25 minutes until cooked through.

Red Pepper and Sausage Wrap   **Serves 2**

2 brown rice tortillas
½ cup red pepper, diced
¼ cup onion, diced
3 eggs, beaten
2 turkey breakfast sausages, cut into small pieces
1 tablespoon olive oil
Salt and pepper – generous pinch

In a frying pan on medium heat the olive oil. Add the sausage and cook until lightly browned. Add the onions and red peppers and cook until onions begin to soften, about 2 minutes. Next, add eggs and salt and pepper. Let eggs sit until they begin to cook slightly and then scramble.

Lightly warm the tortillas and put the egg scramble into the tortillas. Top the eggs with one tablespoon of salsa.

Spinach and Tomato Scramble **Serves 2**

The Parmesan cheese adds a delightful saltiness and tang to this dish.

4 eggs, beaten
1 tablespoon water
2 tablespoons diced onion
¼ tomato, chopped
12 spinach leaves, chopped
1 tablespoon olive oil
Salt and pepper (optional)
Parmesan cheese - or soy Parmesan (optional)

Beat the 4 eggs together with 1 tablespoon water. Preheat the frying pan on medium heat and add 1 tablespoon olive oil. Add onion and cook for about 3 minutes until onions are translucent. Next add eggs, spinach and tomato. Let sit for about 15 seconds and then start to scramble with your spatula. Sprinkle on a small amount of Parmesan cheese, add a pinch of salt and pepper and serve.

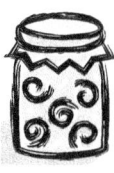 *Spreads and Sauces*

These spreads and sauces contain important nutrients that help to balance your hormones and as well as correct conditions related to estrogen dominance. Estrogen dominant conditions, like fibroid tumors and endometriosis can be a common cause of heavy menstrual bleeding and anemia.

Serve these spreads with rice cakes, crackers, corn bread, or even spread on a banana for a delicious treat.

Fresh Applesauce   Serves 2

2 ½ apples
½ cup fresh apple juice
½ teaspoon cinnamon
½ teaspoon ginger

Peel apples and cut into quarters; remove cores. Combine all ingredients in a food processor. Blend until smooth.

Sesame-Tofu Spread   Serves 4

¼ cup soft tofu
¼ cup raw sesame butter
¼ cup honey

Combine all ingredients in a blender. Serve with rice cakes or crackers.

Lunch and Dinner Recipes

These high-nutrient, healthy lunch and dinner dishes are designed to help prevent and relieve your symptoms. The ingredients do not include red meat, dairy products, or wheat, all of which can worsen your symptoms. Mix and match these dishes as you please. You might combine soups and salads or whole grains, legumes and vegetables for a complete vegetarian emphasis meal. Add chicken, turkey, eggs, or fish for a meat-based meal. Structure each meal depending on your needs for carbohydrates and protein.

The main course dishes are all extremely healthful for women with anemia and estrogen dominant related health issues. You can enjoy these dishes particularly during the second half of your menstrual cycle when your symptoms are worse, but for optimal health and well-being, I recommend their use all month long.

 *Soups*

Split Pea Soup Serves 4

¾ cup split peas
5 cups low-sodium chicken broth
¾ cup carrot, chopped
¾ cup onion, diced
Tamari soy sauce – to taste (optional)

Bring the water to a boil and add the split peas, onion, carrots, and chicken broth. Reduce heat to low and simmer for 50-60 minutes, stirring occasionally. If water begins to cook off add up to an extra cup of water. Add a dash of tamari soy sauce for a saltier flavor.

Black Bean Soup Serves 4

This recipe is easy and makes a delicious, filling soup.

1 can black beans (14 ounce), rinsed
5 cups low-sodium vegetable broth
1 cup onion, diced
⅔ cup carrot, chopped
⅔ cup red pepper, chopped
¼ teaspoon cumin
Tamari soy sauce – to taste (optional)

Bring the water to a boil and add all ingredients. Reduce heat to low and simmer for 30 minutes, stirring occasionally. If water begins to cook off add up to an extra cup of water. Add a dash of tamari soy sauce for a saltier flavor.

Chicken Rice Soup Serves 4-6

Few things make me feel better than a bowl of homemade chicken rice soup. I have an easy tip to add extra flavor to your soup: If you used the meat from a roasted, skin-on chicken you can add some of the skin to the soup while it is cooking. This will add depth and richness to your soup. Remove the skin when the soup has finished cooking.

6 cups low-sodium chicken broth
⅔ cup carrot
1 cup celery, diced
1 cup cooked chicken, diced
⅔ cup onion, diced
⅔ cup brown rice, cooked
Tamari soy sauce – to taste (optional)

Bring water to a boil and add all ingredients. Reduce heat to low and simmer for 30 minutes, stirring occasionally. If water begins to cook off add up to an extra cup of water. Add a dash of tamari soy sauce for a saltier flavor.

Butternut Squash Soup   **Serves 4**

This soup has been a long-time favorite of mine. I adore the light, creamy texture. Adding maple syrup enhances the natural sweetness of the squash.

½ onion, diced
1 cup low-sodium chicken broth
2 cups pureed butternut squash - fresh or frozen (fresh is preferred)
½ teaspoon cinnamon
1½ cups nondairy milk
2 teaspoons maple syrup
1 tablespoon safflower oil
½-¾ teaspoon salt

In a large saucepan heat the oil on medium heat. Add the onion and cook until translucent. Add the butternut squash, chicken broth, cinnamon and salt. Mix well and simmer for 5 minutes. Add nondairy milk and maple syrup. Simmer on low heat for ten minutes. Stir frequently while cooking the soup.

Optional: To make extra creamy, blend the soup when it has finished cooking. Wait for the soup to cool before blending.

 *Salads*

Zingy Watercress Salad   **Serves 4**

I enjoy the refreshing bitterness of watercress. This salad pairs well with green apple. Watercress has a strong flavor and a little goes a long way.

1 cup watercress, coarsely chopped
4 cups butter lettuce (or other soft lettuce), coarsely chopped
2 teaspoons scallions, finely chopped
½ green apple, chopped
1 ounce goat cheese, crumbled
Vinaigrette dressing

In a large bowl toss the watercress, butter lettuce, green onion, and apple together with the vinaigrette dressing (to taste). On top of the salad crumble the goat cheese.

Caesar Salad   **Serves 2-4**

I love Caesar salads. They have been my favorite salad for years! The crispy romaine lettuce and creamy dressing is a perfect match. I like to use anchovies because they are delicious in this salad and also full of healthy anti-inflammatory oils. I prefer the filets packed in olive oil.

1 head of romaine lettuce, chopped – about 6 cups
4 tablespoons light Caesar dressing
4 anchovy filets, chopped
⅔ cup gluten-free croutons
1½ tablespoons grated Parmesan cheese
1 cup roast chicken, cubed (optional)

In a large mixing bowl pour Caesar's dressing over lettuce. Mix well so that leaves are evenly coated with dressing. Add croutons, Parmesan cheese, anchovies, and toss well. Top with roasted chicken and serve.

Classic Spinach Salad   **Serves 4**

My tip for cooking great turkey bacon is to cook it on medium-low heat. It takes a few extra minutes but is definitely worth it!

1 bunch of spinach, approximately 6 cups
4 slices of turkey bacon, cooked crisp and crumbled
2 eggs, sliced or chopped
½ cup red pepper, chopped
¼ red onion, sliced very thin
¾ cup mushrooms, sliced thin
Balsamic Vinaigrette Dressing

In a large bowl place the bacon, egg, red pepper, onion, and mushrooms on top of the spinach. Mix in the dress and toss the salad.

Scrumptious Veggie Salad   **Serves 4-6**

This is one of my favorite salads! It pairs wonderfully with soups and sandwiches.

1 head red lettuce, chopped into bite size pieces
1 large tomato, chopped
2 green onions, sliced
6 mushrooms, sliced
¾ cup kidney beans – canned works well
1 avocado, sliced
¼ cup sunflower seeds
Vinaigrette dressing (to taste)

Combine all ingredients except for avocado in a large salad bowl. Mix in Vinaigrette Dressing and top with avocado slices before serving.

Radicchio and Orange Salad   Serves 4-6

This is a sophisticated and delicious salad. I love salads with "extras" such as fruit or a little bit of goat cheese.

6 cups salad greens
½ radicchio, sliced thin
¼ red onion, sliced very thin
3 ounces goat cheese
1 medium sized orange, peeled and cut into bite size segments
Orange vinaigrette

In a large bowl combine salad greens, radicchio, onion, and oranges. Pour vinaigrette, to taste, over salad and toss. Add goat cheese before serving.

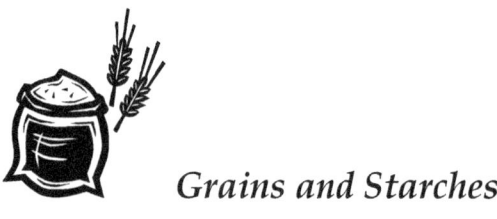

Grains and Starches

Wild Rice   Serves 2

⅔ cup wild rice
2 ½ cups water
½ teaspoon salt

Wash rice with cold water. Combine all ingredients in a cooking pot and bring to a rapid boil. Turn flame to low, cover, and cook without stirring (about 45 minutes) until rice is tender but not mushy. Uncover and fluff with a fork. Cook an additional 5 minutes, and then serve.

Kasha   Serves 4

1 cup kasha (buckwheat groats)
3 ¼ cups water
Pinch of salt

Bring ingredients to a boil, lower heat, and simmer for 25 minutes or until soft. The grains should be fluffy, like rice.

For breakfast, blend in blender with water until creamy. Add almond milk, sesame milk, or sunflower milk, and cinnamon, apple butter, raisins, or berries.

Delicious Baked Sweet Potato   Serves 4

4 sweet potatoes
1 teaspoon olive oil
1 tablespoon flax oil for each potato

Preheat oven to 400° F. Wash the potatoes, then rub with olive oil. Bake for 45 to 60 minutes, or until soft when pierced with a fork. Garnish with flax oil. Honey, maple syrup, or chopped raw pecans may also be used.

Baked Potato **Serves 4**

4 russet or Idaho potatoes
2 teaspoons olive oil
1 tablespoon flax oil for each potato

Preheat oven to 400° F. Wash the potatoes, rub them with olive oil, and bake for 45 to 60 minutes, or until soft when pierced with a fork. Garnish with flax oil. Other garnishes can include chopped green onions, soy cheese, and salsa.

 *Vegetables*

Kale with Lemon   **Serves 4**

Kale is one of my favorite vegetables and it also has terrific health benefits for women since it is a good source of calcium and other essential nutrients like lutein which supports the health of your eyes.

1 bunch of kale
1 lemon, cut into quarters
Soy sauce

Rinse kale well and remove stems. Steam for 5-6 minutes or until leaves wilt and are tender. Dress lightly with soy sauce and lemon juice.

Simple Steamed Cabbage   **Serves 4**

1 small head cabbage, quartered
1 teaspoon chopped parsley
1 teaspoon olive oil
Pinch of salt (optional)

Steam cabbage until tender. Sprinkle with olive oil and parsley.

Jessica's Favorite Broccoli   **Serves 4**

1 pound broccoli
1 tablespoons flax oil
Pinch of salt (optional)
Squeeze of lemon

Cut the broccoli into small flowerets; steam until tender. Squeeze lemon juice over broccoli and add the flax oil. Mix and serve.

Cauliflower with Flax Oil   Serves 4

1 medium head cauliflower
2 tablespoons flax oil
Pinch of salt (optional)

Break the cauliflower into small flowerets. Steam until tender. Toss with flax oil and salt.

Roasted Rosemary Potatoes   Serves 4-6

I love roasted potatoes! This is a wonderful potato recipe that I like to make when I serve roasted chicken.

4 cups red potatoes – about 4 or 5 large red potatoes
1 tablespoon dried rosemary, crushed
3 tablespoons of olive oil
2 garlic cloves, minced
¼ teaspoon pepper (optional)
Pinch of salt

Preheat oven to 400 degrees. Cut potatoes into bite size pieces and put into plastic bag. Add olive oil, rosemary, garlic, and pepper to bag. Close bag and shake to coat all of the potato pieces.

Line a baking tray with foil and put potatoes on to tray. Arrange evenly in one layer. Sprinkle salt onto potatoes and bake for 30-35 minutes until brown and cooked through. During cooking stir the potatoes once if desired.

Honey Carrots **Serves 4**

This is one of my favorite side dishes. The warm honey brings out the natural sweetness of the carrots.

3 cups carrots, sliced thin
1 teaspoon honey
1 teaspoon almond oil
Pinch of salt (optional)

Cut carrots into thin slices and steam for 6-8 minutes, or until tender. Using the same saucepan pour out the cooking water and on low heat add the honey and oil and mix well. Add carrots and mix all ingredients together. Add a pinch of salt before serving.

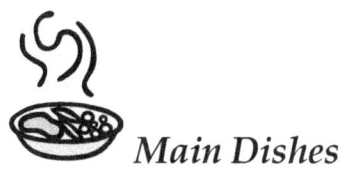 *Main Dishes*

Mega Greens Rice Bowl   **Serves 4**

This dish is a satisfying way to get a large serving of healthy greens. A delicious sauce is Organicville's Island Teriyaki (organicvillefoods.com). Their sauce is made with agave nectar instead of cane sugar.

4 cups kale, cut into bite size pieces (about ½ bunch)
3 cups baby bok choy, chopped
1 cup of white mushrooms, sliced
1 carrot, finely chopped
8 ounces of tofu, cubed
3 cups cooked brown rice - ¾ cup rice per person
Teriyaki sauce – soy sauce - gomasio

Steam the carrots for 4 minutes and then add the kale, bok choy, mushrooms, and tofu. Steam for 5 minutes. Serve in a deep bowl over rice with your choice of sauce.

Good sauces for this dish include teriyaki sauce and soy sauce. A little bit of lemon juice and gomasio also works well.

Teriyaki Tofu Wrap   **Serves 2**

The tofu and teriyaki flavors blend delightfully with the vegetables. This is a light and delicious wrap.

2 brown rice tortillas
6 ounces of baked tofu, cubed or sliced (see recipe)
¼ red pepper, sliced thinly
2 radishes, sliced thinly
1 cup salad greens
½ cup sprouts
2 tablespoons teriyaki sauce

Lightly heat up the tortilla until soft. Layer the vegetables inside and top with the tofu. Lightly pour the sauce on top. Wrap and serve.

Summertime Veggie Pasta   **Serves 4**

This light pasta is one of my favorite dishes to eat during the summer. The pasta and sauce are light but filling. It's a dish that I love to share to share with friends.

1 box quinoa elbow pasta (8 ounce box)
½ onion, diced
2 cans Italian seasoned diced tomatoes
1 can garbanzo beans
1 carrot, shredded
1½ cups cooked Brussels sprouts or broccoli
½ teaspoon dried basil
2 teaspoons olive oil
Pinch of pepper
Pinch of salt (optional)

Cook pasta according to package directions. In a saucepan on medium heat add olive oil and onions. Sautee until onions are translucent. Add remainder of ingredients and bring to a simmer. Cook on low heat for 10 minutes. Combine the cooked noodles with the sauce.

Eggplant Parmesan Serves 4-6

I love eggplant Parmesan. It is a rich and extremely delicious entree. This version, while wonderful, takes a little more time and has a few more steps than most of my entrees. Even though I use substitutions for the cheese, the dish is still very rich and I recommend saving it for a special occasion or party. You will wow your guests with how tasty it is! My favorite cheese alternative is by Follow Your Heart. Their products can be found in health food stores or at followyourheart.com

1 eggplant, cut into ⅓ - ½ inch slices (peeling is optional)
2 eggs, beaten
1 ¼ cups gluten-free breadcrumbs
3 cups of pasta sauce, tomato and basil flavor
8 ounces of mozzarella cheese, shredded
¼ cup Parmesan or soy Parmesan cheese, grated
¼ cup olive oil - divided

Arrange the eggplant slices in a colander or on a rack placed over the sink. Sprinkle all of the slices generously with salt and let stand 30 minutes; the eggplant slices will release water. Rinse and pat dry. Next, dip each slice in the beaten egg and coat with breadcrumbs.

Heat a portion of the olive oil in a skillet over medium heat. Cook the eggplant until golden on each side, about 2-3 minutes. If necessary, reduce the heat to medium-low. Repeat until all of the eggplant is cooked.

Preheat the oven 350°. Arrange half the eggplant slices on the bottom of a lightly oiled baking dish (a 9x9 or 9x12 pan works well). Spread half of the pasta sauce on top. Sprinkle with half of the mozzarella and half of the Parmesan cheese. Repeat with the next layer.

Bake 25-30 minutes or until mixture is bubbly.

The Anemia Cure   73

Parmesan Chicken Pasta **Serves 4**

This dish is a crowd pleaser that I often serve when I have friends over. The Parmesan cheese adds a delightful tanginess that rounds out the dish perfectly.

6 cups gluten-free pasta, cooked
1 ½ cups roasted chicken, cubed
¾ cup diced carrots
¾ cup diced red onion
½ onion, diced
1 small tomato, finely chopped
3 cups broccoli, chopped into bite size pieces
¾ cup chicken broth (recommended) or water
1 teaspoon dried basil
1 tablespoon olive oil
Soy Parmesan cheese or regular, grated (to taste)
Generous pinch of pepper
Pinch of salt (optional)

In a frying pan on medium heat add the olive oil. Add the onion and sauté until onion begin to turn translucent. Add all vegetables except tomatoes and cook for 1-2 minutes. Add chicken broth, chicken, tomatoes, basil, and pepper. Turn heat to low, cover and simmer for 5-7 minutes or until broth has cooked down. Add more broth if needed.

Add the sauce to the pasta. Serve with Parmesan cheese.

Simple Broiled Tuna **Serves 4**

4 fillets of tuna, 4 ounces each
2 teaspoons olive oil
Squeeze of lemon juice
Pinch of salt

Baste the tuna fillets with oil; then sprinkle with lemon juice. Place tuna in a broiler pan and broil until the level of doneness that you prefer (rare or well-done).

Simple Steamed Salmon   **Serves 4**

4 fillets of salmon, 4 ounces each
1 cup water
Squeeze of lemon

Combine water and lemon juice in a steamer. Place salmon fillets in streamer basket. Cook to the level of doneness that you prefer.

Turkey Bolognese   **Serves 2-4**

This dish cooks up quickly and is very satisfying. This is a versatile recipe. You can add all kinds of vegetables and it will taste great.

½ lb. ground turkey
2 cans of diced tomatoes
1 can tomato paste
½ onion, diced
1 carrot, diced
1 zucchini, diced
1 teaspoon basil
1 teaspoon oregano
1 tablespoon olive oil
¼ teaspoon salt (optional)
½ teaspoon black pepper (optional)
Water (optional)

Heat pan on medium and add olive oil. Add onion and sauté until translucent. Add turkey and all herbs and spices. Cook until turkey has browned and cooked thoroughly. Add tomatoes, tomato paste, carrots, and zucchini. Cook on low heat for 12-15 minutes. If sauce is too thick add a small amount of water until desired consistency is reached. Serve over brown rice spaghetti.

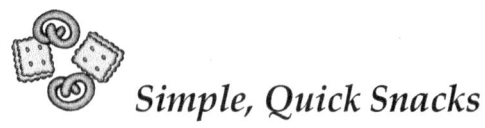 *Simple, Quick Snacks*

Trail Mix   **Makes ¾ cup**

¼ cup raw unsalted pumpkin seeds
¼ cup raw unsalted sunflower seeds
¼ cup raisins

Combine and store in a container in the refrigerator. This trail mix is very high in essential fatty acids, calcium, magnesium, and iron. I use it for a snack food to replace stressful and unhealthy sugar-based sweets and chocolate. It is a great mix to take on trips, and I eat it often for breakfast.

Rice Cakes with Nut Butter and Jam   **Serves 2**

4 unsalted rice cakes
2 tablespoons raw almond butter
2 tablespoons fruit preserves (no sugar added)

Spread rice cakes with almond butter and fruit preserves for a quick snack.

Herbal tea makes a good accompaniment.

Rice Cakes with Tuna Fish   **Serves 2**

4 unsalted rice cakes
4 ounces tuna fish
2 teaspoons low-calorie mayonnaise

Spread rice cakes with tuna fish and mayonnaise.

This is an excellent high-protein, high-carbohydrate snack.

Apple with Almond Butter   **Serves 2**

1 apple, sliced
1 tablespoon raw almond butter

Spread almond butter on thin apple slices.

Banana with Sesame Butter   **Serves 2**

1 banana, halved
1 tablespoon raw sesame butter

Spread sesame butter on each half of a ripe banana.

5

Putting Your Program Together

I have shared with you a self-care program to help heal and relieve your symptoms of anemia. My program will not only help you to solve this issue but should also create a great improvement in your overall health and well-being.

I usually recommend beginning any self-care program slowly while you get used to the changes in lifestyle. People differ in their ability to adjust to major lifestyle changes. Though some of my patients like to eliminate their old, unhealthy habits as quickly as possible, many other women find such rapid changes in long-term habits too stressful. Find the pace that works for you.

Enjoy the program. I always tell my patients to regard their self-care program as an enjoyable adventure. The exercises and stress-reduction techniques should give you a sense of renewed energy and well-being. The menus and food selections I've recommended in this book provide you with an opportunity to try delicious and healthful new recipes and meal plans.

As you do the program, don't set up unrealistic or overly strict expectations for yourself. You don't have to be perfect to get great results. Just follow the guidelines of the program as best you can and as your schedule permits.

It is not a major issue if you forget to take your vitamins occasionally or don't have time to exercise on a particular day. Don't be discouraged if you can't follow the dietary recommendations on vacations, holidays, and birthdays. Periodically review the guidelines outlined in this book and continue to adapt your lifestyle to the healthful suggestions that I've shared with you from my years of medical practice. Over time you will notice many beneficial changes.

Be your own feedback system. Your body will tell you if you are on the right track and if what you are doing is making you feel better. It will also tell you if your current diet and emotional stresses are worsening your symptoms. Remember that even moderate changes in your habits can make significant differences.

The Anemia Workbook

Fill out the workbook section of this book. The workbook questionnaires will help you determine which areas in your life have contributed the most to your symptoms and need the most improvement. Review the workbook every month or two as you follow the self-help program. The workbook will help you see the areas in which you are making the most progress, with both symptom relief and the adoption of healthier lifestyle habits. The workbook can help give you feedback in an organized and easy-to-use manner.

Diet and Nutritional Supplements

I recommend that you make all nutritional changes gradually. Many women find breakfast the easiest meal to change because it is simple and often eaten at home. To change your other meals and snacks, periodically review the list of foods to eliminate and foods to emphasize. Each month, pick a few foods that you are willing to eliminate from your diet. Try in their place the foods that help prevent and relieve heavy menstrual bleeding. The recipes and menus that I have included in my book should be very helpful, use the meal plans as guidelines while you restructure your diet to suit your needs.

Vitamins, minerals, essential fatty acids, and herbal supplements can help complete your nutritional needs and speed up the healing process. I have found the use of these nutritional supplements to be a very beneficial, even essential, part of your program.

Conclusion

I want to inspire you that you have a tremendous ability to heal and that you can enjoy radiant health and well-being. By having access to the self-care resources contained in this book, you can play a major role in creating your own state of great health. Practice the beneficial self-care techniques that I've outlined in this book. Follow good nutritional habits, exercise, and practice stress-reduction techniques regularly.

By combining these beneficial principles of self-care, you can enjoy the same wonderful results that my patients and I have had in healing anemia.

Love,

Dr. Susan

About Susan Richards, M.D.

Dr. Susan Richards is one of the foremost authorities in the fields of family medicine and alternative medicine. Dr. Richards has successfully treated many thousands of patients emphasizing alternative health and integrative medicine in her clinical practice. Her mission is to provide her patients with safe and effective alternative therapies to greatly enhance their health and well-being.

A graduate of Northwestern University Feinberg School of Medicine, she has served on the clinical faculty of Stanford University School of Medicine and taught in their Division of Family and Community Medicine.

Her Facebook page, Dr. Susan's Healthy Living, has over one million followers. She is also an ordained minister and her ministry receives over a million prayer requests for healing each year.

NOTES

NOTES